LOW CARB HIGH FAT

*The Ultimate Guide to
Lose Weight and Eat More*

FREE BONUSES

As Promised Here is Your Guide To Low Carb Diets

CLICK HERE To Get Your Copy

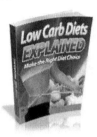

If You Want Free Best Selling Kindle Books Delivered To You Weekly

CLICK HERE

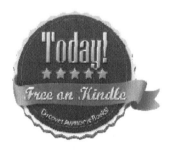

Table of contents

Introduction

I want to thank you and congratulate you for downloading the book, *"Low Carb/High Fat Diet: The Ultimate Guide to Lose Weight and Eat More"*.

This book contains proven steps and strategies on how to shed those excess pounds without starving yourself at the same time.

This diet will be unlike any of the other diets you've probably already tried. Most diets are based on deprivation; the idea that if you deprive yourself of food you'll lose the weight. Now that science has proven that theory to be highly inaccurate, it's time to embark on something entirely new (well, sort of).

The Low Carb/High Fat diet addresses this all important issue of how to lose weight without having to starve yourself. In addition, you'll find that weight you will be able to eat much more food than you ever thought you could.

There is a common misconception in the world right now. It's the idea that we all struggle with losing weight. But that's not really the case with most diets. People have seen great success in losing those extra pounds, where they have failed, however is in keeping it off. With the Low Carb/High Fat diet, you'll be learning an entirely new way to eat so that part of the diet is focused on learning how to eat for life.

Instead of eating for a few weeks or months to lose the weight and returning to your old habits, you'll learn how to eat for life. This will mean that this could very well be the very last diet you'll ever have to try. I'll bet that's worth quite a bit to you and probably a lot of other people.

I hope you can find great benefit in the knowledge you'll find in the following pages. It is our hope that by following it you'll find a completely way to see food, enjoy it, and use it in a way that can improve your life in many ways.

Thanks again for downloading this book, I hope you enjoy it!

CHAPTER 1

An Insight Into the Low Carb and High Fat Diet

I f you've found your way to this book then there is a pretty good chance that you're interested in one of the most efficient ways to lose weight. Considering this objective, there are numerous ways you could choose to go about achieving your objective. Clearly some will be more effective than others. However, one of the most productive and efficient ways to do this is through the Low Carb/High Fat Diet, which encourages you to reduce your consumption of carbohydrates and increase the amount of fats at the same time. While this method seems quite simple, the method has been gaining in popularity over the years attracting a large number of people and motivating them to follow it.

This chapter of the book will give you a balanced perspective into the Low Carb/High Fat diet and what you should know about it. It is important for you to understand that our general objective is to help you to understand the basic fundamentals of the diet and what is expected of you to make it a success. Once that groundwork is laid, we will be able to move on to more practical steps and guidelines to follow in the following chapters. With all of that said, let's begin.

As the name suggests, it is a regular eating routine, which consists of consuming foods with a high fat content along with a smaller percentage of carbohydrates. While you may not have heard of the low car/high fat diet before, chances are you've heard of it by its more popular term; The Atkins Diet.

The diet is based on an extensive body of research that has been done over the past eight years. As a result, it has been recommended as one of the most effective solutions for weight loss. This is one of the reasons why you can walk into any bookstore and find so many books that have been written on it. In fact, over the years, with its increasing popularity, it has become a global phenomenon.

There may be many reasons why the diet is so popular but the most common reason is because it's effective. It's a nutrition program that has consistently gotten results that make it worth the extra effort put forth to do it well. Through several research studies (which we will link you to later in the book) it is proven effective not just in weight loss but in improving the blood pressure and cholesterol levels than many other similar weight loss programs.

So, what is the low carb/high fat diet?

The thought behind this type of nutrition program is that you can eat as much protein ad fat as you want but you need to avoid any foods that are high in carbs. That's the simple and most basic explanation of this type of diet so we need to dig a little deeper to understand why this is so effective in helping people to lose weight.

The Studies

Over the past dozen or so years there have been more than 20 studies (http://authoritynutrition.com/23-studies-on-low-carb-and-low-fat-diets/) that have shown that low-carb diets are an effective tool for weight loss. Not only is it an easier program to follow, there are some highly desirable benefits to our overall health as an added bonus.

The diet was the brainchild of a physician by the name of Dr. Robert C. Atkins, who introduced the low carb diet in his book in the early 70s. Since that time, the diet has become one of the most popular diet programs ever in our recorded history.

Initially believed to be unhealthy by most health professionals because of its high saturated fat content, it was a controversial subject for quite some time. However, their beliefs lead to a common misconception that it would raise the Low-density lipoprotein (LDL) or "bad" cholesterol in the body. However, recent studies (The Meta-analysis of prospective cohort studies evaluating the association of saturated fat with cardiovascular disease and the association of dietary, circulating, and supplement fatty acids with coronary risk) have shown that in many cases fatty acids are not as dangerous as many people had once believed.

To date, the diet has been put through an expensive battery of tests and has undergone careful scrutiny and has been shown to contribute more to weight loss than the previously supported low-fat diets. The studies have also taken note that those on The Atkins Diet have seen improvements in their blood sugar levels (HDL), triglycerides, and other essential health markers.

Despite the fact that the diet is high in fat, in many cases it was noted that the Atkins Diet did not raise the LDL cholesterol levels. Although in some cases it was known to happen in a small subset of individuals, the vast majority of them saw an actual reduction of the LDL numbers.

What Makes the Low Carb/High Fat Diet So Effective?

By and large, the most likely reason that the diet is so effective in reducing weight is that when the consumption of carbs is reduced and the proteins are increased the natural appetite decreases and the dieter will naturally consume fewer calories overall without the added calorie counting.

So far, all the evidence proves that it is safe to suggest that the Low Carb/High Fat diet is one of the most effective solutions for weight loss in many people. This is the primary reason why we have seen so many books that have been written to promote this unique and special diet.

CHAPTER 2

The Phases of the Low Carb/High Fat Diet

W hen practiced in the right manner, this diet can be divided into four main phases, which when followed correctly will yield the best results.

Phase 1 (Induction): This phase is your initiation phase into the program. It is important to note that this part of the diet does not represent the whole diet plan. Many in the past have been confused with this fact and have viewed the program as a failure because they have never moved beyond this phase. However, Induction is only the first of four transitions you will go through to get the best results.

The Induction phase has two main objectives:

A. To get your body to switch from burning primary carbohydrates (usually stored in the form of glucose) to burning your fat stores for energy.
B. To kick-start your weight loss.

To get your body to burn more fat, this phase requires you to limit your carbs to only 20 grams a day. In addition, you want to limit your carb intake to vegetables that are rich in antioxidants, minerals, vitamins and other essential nutrients including fiber.

While it is not necessary to start the diet in the induction phase, it is strongly recommended because it is a faster and more efficient means of turning your body into a fat-burning machine.

For most people, it will be good to remain on Phase I for a minimum of two weeks. The exception to this would be those who would do not have a lot of weight to lose and find it easy to shed those excess pounds quickly. For those people, you can move on to Phase 2 after only one week.

The Rules: Most people will be amazed at the amount of weight loss you'll see in the induction phase but there will be others who will find it hard to kick-start their body into the fat burning machine they want. Your body will find its own pace to shed those pounds but in order to get the best results there are a few rules that you should keep in mind. By sticking to the guidelines listed below, you'll soon that you're on your way to the best results.

1. Make sure you eat a minimum of three regular size meals every day. Avoid the tendency to skip meals or to go more than six hours without eating. If you're not hungry at mealtime, eat a small snack.

2. It is important for you to consume a minimum of 4-6 oz (115-175 grams) of protein. This can include meats like poultry, beef, lamb, pork, and veal. It can also include seafood, both fish and shellfish, or dairy – eggs, cheese. You can also incorporate a number of high protein vegetables like soybeans, edamame, lentils, broccoli, peas, asparagus, pumpkin seeds, or mung bean sprouts.

3. Don't be afraid to use healthy fats. Feel free to add real butter, olive oil or a high-oleic sunflower oil but don't go overboard. Try to limit your consumption to 1 tablespoon of oil for your salad or other vegetables. When cooking just use enough oil to ensure that your food doesn't burn or you can use a cooking spray instead.

4. Never eat more than 20 grams of net carbs a day but make sure that 12-15 grams come from your vegetables. This equates to approximately six cup of salad or two cups of vegetables a day.

5. Get yourself a carb counter, this will prevent you from guessing about the amount of carbs you're eating. Remember, vegetable carbs can vary greatly so you need to be sure.

6. Only eat the foods on your list. (Included later in the chapter)

7. On average, with the exception of cottage cheese or ricotta, you can have up to 4 ounces of cheese per day, 10

black olives or up to 20 green olives, a half an avocado (look for those with the blackish skin), 1 oz. of sour cream, and 3 Tablespoons of cream, lemon or lime juice. While these foods are okay to eat, you still must include their carb count into your daily 20 gram allowance.

8. Try to avoid sugars but to satisfy your sweet tooth, consider sweetening your foods with Splenda, Sweet 'N Low, Stevia, or Xylitol. Do not go over three packs a day and consider each package a 1 gram of carbs. While these sweeteners do not contain carbs themselves, they are often packaged with fillers that do.

9. You can also satisfy your cravings for sweets with a sugar-free gelatin desert or up to two Atkins shakes or bars. (Make sure that you pick one that is coded for Induction.

10. Drink at least 8 oz of approved beverages. These include water, herbal teas, or coffee to avoid dehydration and an imbalance in your electrolytes. You can also include two cups of broth; drink one in the morning and the other one in the afternoon.

11. Don't assume that a food is low carb. Always read the labels to make sure.

12. Take at least one iron-free multivitamin and an omega-e supplement for fatty-acids.

13. Eating for many people is a habit; it is essential that you analyze your cravings for food. Know the difference between eating because your body craves sustenance and eating because it's a habit. When you eat, stop when you're satisfied. If in doubt – push the plate away and

wait ten minutes, then drink a glass of water. If you still want to eat after that then you're not full.

14. When you're eating out, keep on the look out for hidden carbs. You'll find them in foods like gravy (made with flour or cornflower), salad dressings usually contain sugars, and fried foods often are breaded. All of these foods are not allowed on the diet.

It may take you a little while to master the rules but if followed correctly, you'll quickly begin to see the results in weight loss as you pass through the induction period.

Phase 2 (Balancing): The second phase of the diet allows you to make a few additions to your meals. Not only will you be allowed to add nuts and seeds but you can also include a minimal amount of fruits and low carb veggies into your meal plan.

This phase helps you to start climbing up the Carb Ladder by gradually introducing different foods into your meal plans in 5-carb increments. It is in this phase that the bulk of your weight loss will occur. Unlike in the first phase, where you had a definite time frame to stay on the program, you will remain in this phase until you only have ten pounds or less remaining to reach your target weight. Of course, you can transition to Phase 3 sooner if you find that your weight is dropping off too fast and you want to slow down the pace.

This phase is called balancing because it is the point where you will be able to adapt your eating routine to find the balance of food that works best for your body.

There is a variety of foods you'll be able to add and test out until you can find a healthy balance that'll work for you. During Phase 1 you gained a little weight loss momentum so it's important that the switch can help you to maintain that momentum and continue the process through finding your personal carb balance (the point where your intake of carbs balances with the amount of energy you spend).

The beginning of Phase 3 will be a testing ground from which you build on. In the Induction Phase you were restricted to consuming only 20 grams of carbs a day, but in the balancing phase you'll begin by making small 5-gram increases to your carb intake. You will monitor your progress until you find your personal carb balance, which could level off at anywhere from 30 to 80 grams of carbs every day. This personal balance point will be different for each person, as it will be determined by such factors as your activity level, age, gender, hormones, and a number of other things.

Your goal is to find a sustainable way of eating that will continue to help you to lose weight without diminishing your level of energy. This is where you can begin to see the benefits of the Atkins program. Rather than being tied to a finite list of foods you can eat, you'll be free to dine out, prepare meals for special occasions or just enjoy some of your own favorite foods without breaking in predetermined diet rules.

The rules in Phase 1 were to give you basic guidelines to follow to lose weight but now you're going to start making these incremental changes to determine what is called your Carb Tolerance. It is a diet that puts you in control. You're in search of the number of carbs you can consume and still be able to lose weight. At this point, the differences between Phase 1 and Phase 2 will be minor but you'll still need to do the following:

- Count and monitor your carb consumption daily.
- Eat only the recommended options of proteins and fats on the approved list (see in next chapter).
- Drink at least eight glasses of approved fluids every day.
- Ensure that you're getting enough salt in your diet. (This quantity will change with everyone. Those who are on diuretics will have to adjust their diet accordingly). This is in order to avoid experiencing extreme fatigue or other symptoms that may occur when you boost your metabolism to burn more fat.
- Continue with your multivitamins and omega-3 supplements.

You'll still need to avoid the added sugars and make sure that you schedule in enough meals and snacks throughout the day.

Just remember to introduce new carbs in your diet one at a time following the Carb Ladder. This is usually done at weekly intervals but some people prefer to test out these new foods for a longer period of time so you can extend into 2 weeks on each food or even longer.

As you introduce each food, gauge its impact on your body by monitoring your level of energy and the amount of weight you're losing. This has to be carefully done. For example, in week 1 you introduce walnuts to your diet. Monitor your body's response and then move on to the next food item. Adding walnuts is not the same as adding nuts to your diet as each type of nut will create a different response, so they will need to be added one at a time; walnuts one week, almonds the next, peanuts, the following or cashews the next. As you can see, testing the results of each of these foods could take quite a long time to do.

Avoid the Carb Creep

While this phase of the diet will naturally grant you more freedom you'll still need to be extremely careful to make sure that you avoid what is called the 'carb creep.' This occurs as you gradually begin to add these new foods to your diet. You may find that you're suddenly consuming far more carbs than you thought. And because of the new freedom you may become more complacent about monitoring your carb intake and suddenly your weight loss hits a block in the road. To avoid this from happening to you, always remember to monitor and track your carbs and portion sizes for everything you eat.

How to Know When You're Ready for Phase 3

There are several ways to know if you're ready to move on to Phase 3 in your Low Carb/High Fat diet. The most obvious point is if you're within 10 pounds of your target weight you're ready to move on. But in reality, everyone is different so here are a few more points to consider:

1. You're taking in around 50 grams of carbs a day, have already introduced the Phase 2 foods, and you're continuing to lose weight without those nasty cravings or hunger pangs.

2. If you've reached a point where your weight loss has stalled and you have more than 10 pounds to go but you

don't have cravings for certain foods and you don't experience undue hunger pangs. If however, you're still having cravings and hunger, you need to remain in Phase 2 until they have vanished.

3. If you were successful with weight loss in Phase 1 but in Phase 2 your progress has been slow; your cravings and hunger have increased or you've seen a weight gain instead of loss, you may have developed what is called a carb tolerance and have surpassed your carb balance point. At this point you need to boost up your activity level and see if that doesn't improve your weight loss results. If it does, feel free to move on to Phase 3.

Keep in mind that the closer you stick to the plan the more effective the program will be. But don't be surprised to see some occasional variations in your results. This is a testing phase so as you add each new food you'll see some variations in your progress.

Phase 3 (Fine Tuning):

In the third phase of the diet, the pre-maintenance or fine tuning phase, you'll be making the new diet program your own. This phase is very important as it is setting the stage for a lifetime of new healthy eating habits with nutrition as your primary goal.

At this point, you are now within 5-10 pounds of your target weight and you're ready to perfect your new habits that you will carry on into the future. Your weight loss at this point will be gradual but it will help you to be able to transition to your new way of eating, which will be instrumental in maintaining your weight loss from this point on.

How it Works

If done correctly, you'll be able to add a little more carbs to your diet and still be able to shed those last few pounds. During the last phase you were increasing your carb intake in increments of 5 grams. At this point you will be able to boost that up to 10 grams increments. These increases can continue as long as you're able to lose weight. Ideally, you want your weight loss to be less than a pound a week.

Maintain this routine until you have reached your target weight and can maintain it for one month. Your goal is to find your optimum level of carbohydrates you can take in and neither gain or lose weight from it.

Even though you've almost reached your target weight, you still may find yourself frustrated from time to time. Here are a few tips to keep you on the straight and narrow.

- As you're adding those old foods back into your diet, those old cravings may resurface. You'll have to identify the foods that may be sabotaging your progress and eliminate them from your meals for a few days. If the cravings go away, try to reintroduce them again at a later date but if the cravings return, you may want to remove them from your diet permanently.
- You may find that your weight loss has plateaued. When that happens you need to make sure that you've hit a true plateau before you make a decision. This means going

back and making sure that you've followed everything exactly right and that you haven't missed a beat. If it's a real plateau, then cut your carb intake by 10 grams and maintain until your body is ready to break through and start responding.

- It is easy to assume that your carb tolerance level is actually a plateau, the body's responses can be very similar. To distinguish between the two cut back on your carbs by 10 grams for a week or more. If your weight loss kicks in again, go up only 5 grams instead of 10 until you reach your target weight.

If you follow all of these steps and you've reached your target weight, you're ready to move on to Phase 4.

Phase 4: Lifetime Maintenance

The final phase can be called the hallelujah phase. It's the point you've been working for all along; you've reached your target weight and now you need to focus on how to adapt your eating habits to maintain it.

In most cases, failure of other diets is not in being able to shed the pounds but in being able to keep it off. This challenge can be avoided if you know how to apply the strategies outlined in Phase 4 of the low carb/high fat plan.

For the most part, the foods you've been eating all long won't change very much. However, there were likely some foods that you tried previously to reintroduce without success that your body will now be better equipped to handle. This is the time when you can retest the waters to see if you're ready for the new changes.

This is a phase that is going to change your life forever. Unlike the other phases of the program, phase 4 represents an ongoing effort that will eventually become your permanent way of eating. If done correctly, it will help you to maintain control of your weight and teach you how to adjust your carb intake as your tolerance levels change throughout your life. If followed correctly, you'll never have to go on another diet again.

The Rules: Now that you've reached your goal weight the only way to maintain it is to follow the rules.

- Stick to your carb tolerance level. This is the threshold that has helped you maintain your weight for a month in the final part of Phase 3.
- Continue to consume a minimum of 12-15 grams of carbs in the form of vegetables.
- Continue to eat 4-6 ounces of cooked protein at every meal.
- Eat no more than two servings of fruit every day.
- View fat as an important part of your daily diet.
- Balance your carbs with fat and protein to keep your blood sugars level.
- Always drink lots of water and other noncaloric beverages.
- Decrease carbs when you're not active/increase when you are active.
- Remember the difference between real hunger and habitual eating.
- Continue to weigh yourself every week.
- Never allow your weight to go up more than 5 pounds without making an adjustment.
- Continue to add new foods to the program one-at-a-time.

- Stay physically active
- Prepare your food ahead of time, measuring portions carefully.
- Always read labels on the foods you eat; never assume you know.
- Keep on the watch for carb creep.
- Plan for any occasional changes in your diet (even if it is only temporary).

What You've Learned so Far

Throughout the program you have developed some valuable skills that you will be able to use to keep your weight under control. Think about these new skills you have developed.

- Through each phase you've taught your body how to properly use carbs building up your tolerance as you go.
- You've identified foods that you know your body won't be able to tolerate and found ways to navigate around them.
- You've learned which foods you can only take in small doses and which ones you need to avoid altogether.
- You've learned how to identify true hunger as opposed to cravings and how to respond to each one in the right way.
- You've discovered how to trade high-carb foods for low-carb ones and still be satisfied.
- You've found a program that actually works and helps you to look good physically and feel good emotionally.

This final phase of the program is really not a phase in the same way as the other three phases. The transition to this point should be seamless, so there should be no anxiety associated with it. As long as you follow the acceptable foods list found in the following chapter, you'll be able to remain in this phase successfully for months and even years to come.

You'll still need to keep a close watch on your weight gain (it will happen) but now you are armed with the tools to keep it from getting out of control. As you get older, you'll notice that your body will change and you'll need to readjust your eating habits once again. This is perfectly normal and with the things you've learned in this program, you'll quickly readjust and get on with your life rather than spending your time on those on again off again diets that have failed nearly everyone that's tried them.

CHAPTER 3

_____

Acceptable Foods to Eat

oing through this diet will be unlike any other diet you
have ever had to follow. You won't be counting calories
you'll be counting carbs. You won't need to concern
yourself with fat grams or spend time calculating proteins and
what nots. Your only concern will be in controlling your carbs
and staying within the recommended portion sizes.

Now that you have a basic understanding about the diet, you
can look at the program in more detail. But even before that can
happen, it is extremely important to know and understand how
the foods you choose will work together to help you lose weight.
We'll discuss these acceptable foods in detail in this chapter.

As you go through each phase of the program, your food choices
will vary. In the beginning, your carb limitations will be very
strict. Your options for food choices will be restrictive on a
number of levels but once you advance on through each of the

successive phases, you'll be able to have a little bit more freedom to choose the kinds of foods you wish to eat. Remember, you want to keep your carb count down to no more than 20 in Phase 1 of the program, and 12-15 grams of those carbs should be coming from low carb vegetables. Still you want to make sure that you have enough to eat so start by choosing the type of foods that have the lowest amount of carbs. That way, you can eat more of them to keep you sustained.

Phase I Induction Acceptable Foods

From the very beginning of the Induction Phase, you are free to eat all types of meat, fish, shellfish, and choose from a wide selection of vegetables. When you look at the acceptable list, you should see that the meat and fish options have 0 carbs while the vegetables on your list have only trace amounts of carbs.

Use the list below to help you choose the type of foods you can eat as you build up a nutritional meal pan. Of course in the following chapters we will give you some definitive recipes to follow however, if you plan to stick to this program for a long time, you'll quickly tire of eating the same things over and over again. Knowing how to pick the right foods and mix up your diet a bit will give you the motivation to stick to it for a longer period of time.

Fish	Serving size	Net Carbs
Cod	100 grams	0
Flounder	100 grams	0
Halibut	100 grams	0
Herring	100 grams	0

Mackerel	100 grams	0
Salmon	100 grams	0
Sardines	100 grams	0
Seabass	100 grams	0
Sole	100 grams	0
Tuna	100 grams	0
Trout	100 grams	0

Fowl	**Serving size**	**Net Carbs**
Chicken	100 grams	0
Duck	100 grams	0
Goose	100 grams	0
Pheasant	100 grams	0
Turkey	100 grams	0

Eggs	**Serving size**	**Net Carbs**
Deviled	2 eggs	3 grams
Fried	1 medium	0.6 grams
Hardboiled	1 medium	0.6 grams
Omelet	2 medium	1.2 grams (10 grs butter)
Poached	1 medium	0.6 grams
Scrambled	2 medium	1.9 grams (15 ml milk)

Vegetables	**Serving size**	**Net Carbs**
Alfalfa Sprouts	236 grams	0.4 grams
Artichoke	¼ medium artichoke	4.0 grams
Artichoke Hearts	1 can	1.0 grams
Arugula	118 grams	0.2 grams
Asparagus	6 spears	2.4 grams

Aubergine	118 grams	1.8 grams
Avocados	1	3.5 grams
Bamboo Shoots	236 grams	1.1 grams
Bok Choy	236 grams	0.8 grams
Broccoflower	118 grams	1.4 grams
Broccoli	236 grams	0.8 grams
Brussell Sprouts	59 grams	2.4 grams
Cabbage	118 grams	2.0 grams
Cabbage Red	75 grams	2.0 grams
Cauliflower	118 grams	1.0 grams
Celeriac	80 grams	3.5 grams
Celery	1 stalk	0.8 grams
Chicory	118 grams	0.6 grams
Chives	1 Tablespoon	0.1 grams
Collard Greens	118 grams	4.2 grams
Courgette	118 grams	2.0 grams
Cucumber	118 grams	1.0 grams
Daikon Radish	118 grams	1.0 grams
Endive	118 grams	0 grams
Escarole Lettuce	118 grams	0 grams
Fennel	236 grams	3.6 grams
Hearts of Palm	1 heart	0.7 grams
Iceberg Lettuce	118 grams	0.1 grams
Jicama	118 grams	2.5 grams
Kale	118 grams	2.4 grams
Kohlrabi	118 grams	4.6 grams
Leeks	59 grams	1.7 grams

Low Carb High Fat

Mangetout	80 grams	3.4 grams
Mesclun	30 grams	0.5 grams
Mung Bean Sprout	50 grams	2.1 grams
Mushrooms	118 grams	1.2 grams
Okra	118 grams	2.4 grams
Olives	1 olive	0.5 grams
Onion	59 grams	2.8 grams
Parsley	1 Tablespoon	0.1 gram
Peas	118 grams (in the pod)	3.4 grams
Peppers	118 grams	2.3 grams
Pumpkin	59 grams	2.4 grams
Radicchio	118 grams	0.7 grams
Radishes	10 radishes	0.9 grams
Rhubarb	118 grams	1.7 grams
Rocket	20 grams	0.4 grams
Romaine Lettuce	118 grams	0.2 grams
Sauerkraut	118 grams	1.2 grams
Spaghetti Squash	118 grams	2.0 grams
Spinach	118 grams	0.2 grams
Spring Onion	25 grams	1.2 grams
Summer Squash	118 grams	2.0 grams
Swiss Chard	118 grams	1.8 grams
Tomato	1 raw tomato	4.3 grams
Turnip	118 grams	2.2 grams
Water Chestnuts	118 grams	6.9 grams

Low Carb High Fat

Herbs	Serving Size	Net Carbs
Basil	1 teaspoon	0 grams
Bay Leaf	1 teaspoon	0 grams
Coriander	1 teaspoon	0 grams
Dill	1 teaspoon	0 grams
Lemongrass	1 teaspoon	0 grams
Marjoram	1 teaspoon	0 grams
Mint	1 teaspoon	0 grams
Oregano	1 teaspoon	0 grams
Parsley	1 teaspoon	0.1 grams
Rosemary	1 teaspoon	0 grams
Sage	1 teaspoon	0 grams
Thyme	1 teaspoon	0 grams

Meat	Serving Size	Net Carbs
Bacon	1 slice	0.1 grams
Beef	200 grams	0 grams
Ham	1 slice	0 grams
Lamb	1 pound	0 grams
Mutton	1 pound	0 grams
Pork	1 pound	0 grams
Steak	1 pound	0 grams
Venison	1 pound	0 grams

Shellfish	Serving Size	Net Carbs
Crabmeat	118 grams	0 grams
Mussels	236 grams	5.5 grams
Octopus	100 grams	4.4 grams

Oysters	6 medium	3.3 grams
Shrimp	100 grams	1 grams
Squid	100 grams	3 grams

Spices	Serving Size	Net Carbs
Allspice	1 teaspoon	0 grams
Cardamon	1 teaspoon	0 grams
Cayenne	1 teaspoon	0 grams
Celery Salt	1 teaspoon	0 grams
Chili Powder	1 teaspoon	0 grams
Cinnamon	1 teaspoon	0 grams
Cumin	1 teaspoon	0 grams
Garlic	1 teaspoon	0 grams
Ginger	1 teaspoon	0 grams
Mustard Powder	1 teaspoon	0 grams
Nutmeg	1 teaspoon	0 grams
Paprika	1 teaspoon	0 grams
Saffron	1 teaspoon	0 grams
Tumeric	1 teaspoon	0 grams

Cheeses	Serving Size	Net Carbs
Bleu Cheese	30 grams	0.4 grams
Brie	30 grams	0.1 grams
Cheddar Cheese	30 grams	0.4 grams
Cream Cheese	30 grams	0.8 grams
Feta Cheese	30 grams	1.2 grams
Goat Cheese	30 grams	0.3 grams
Gouda Cheese	30 grams	0.6 grams

Mozzarella Cheese	30 grams	0.6 grams
Parmesan Cheese	30 grams	0.9 grams
Swiss Cheese	30 grams	1.0 grams

Fats	Serving Size	Net Carbs
Butter	1 teaspoon	0 grams
Canola Oil	1 teaspoon	0 grams
Coconut Oil	1 Tablespoon	0 grams
Grapeseed Oil	1 Tablespoon	0 grams
Mayonnaise	1 Tablespoon	0 grams
Olive Oil	1 Tablespoon	0 grams

Tofu	Serving Size	Net Carbs
Almond Milk	225 ml	1.0 grams
Quom Burgers	1 burger	4.0 grams
Quom Chicken Cutlet	1 cutlet	3.0 grams
Quom Roast	115 grams	4.0 grams
Seltan	1 piece	2.0 grams
Shirataki Soya Noodles	90 grams	1.0 grams
Soya Cheese	30 grams	2.0 grams
Soya Milk	225 ml	1.2 grams
Tempeh	85 grams	3.3 grams
Firm	115 grams	2.5 grams
Sausage	55 grams	2.5 grams
Vegan Cheese	30 grams	6.0 grams
Veggie Burger	1 burger	2.0 grams

Phase Two Acceptable Foods

When you go to Phase Two of the program, you will simply maintain the same foods and serving sizes as on the Phase One list with a few new additions. In this Phase you will also have more freedom and variety as you are able to up your carb intake by an additional 5 daily net carbs per week. This will allow you to expand your options by including nuts, seeds, and berries in your diet. With these new foods in your program you can much more easily pack a few snacks to get you through the day.

Nuts	Serving Size	Net Carbs
Almonds	30 nuts	5.2 grams
Almond Butter	1 Tablespoon	2.5 grams
Brazil Nuts	10 nuts	4.0 grams
Cashew Butter	1 Tablespoon	4.1 grams
Coconut Shredded	4 Tablespoons	1.3 grams
Hazelnuts	12 nuts	0.5 grams
Hulled Pumpkin Seeds	2 Tablespoons	2.0 grams
Hulled Sunflower Seeds	2 Tablespoons	1.1 grams
Macadamias	12 nuts	4.0 grams
Macadamia Butter	1 Tablespoon	2.5 grams
Peanuts	22 nuts	1.5 grams
Peanut Butter	1 Tablespoon	2.4 grams
Pecans	10 nuts	3.0 grams
Pine Kernels	2 Tablespoons	1.7 grams
Pistachios	50 nuts	5.0 grams
Sesame Seeds	2 Tablespoons	1.6 grams

Soy Nuts	2 Tablespoons	2.7 grams
Sunflower Seed Butter	1 Tablespoon	1.0 grams
Tahini	1 Tablespoon	0.8 grams
Walnuts	14 nuts	5.0 grams

Fruit	Serving Size	Net Carbs
Blackberries	36 grams	2.7 grams
Blueberries	59 grams	5.1 grams
Cantaloupe	59 grams	3.5 grams
Cherries	39 grams	2.8 grams
Cranberries	25 grams	2.0 grams
Gooseberries	75 grams	4.4 grams
Raspberries	59 grams	3.6 grams
Strawberries	59 grams	2.6 grams

Cheeses (these are new cheeses not on the list for Phase 1)

Cottage Cheese	100 grams	2.8 grams
Greek Yogurt	115 grams	3.5 grams
Natural Yogurt	115 grams	5.5 grams
Ricotta Cheese	180 grams	5.7 grams

Phase Three Acceptable Foods

By the time you reach Phase Three, you should have mastered the acceptable food list. With just a few more additions, you should have developed the skill of choosing the right foods to eat and the right portions. Now you can introduce legumes, fruit, and more higher carb veggies into your meal plan.

Low Carb High Fat

Legumes	Serving Size	Net Carbs
Black Beans	118 grams	12.9 grams
Chickpeas	118 grams	16.2 grams
Great Northern Beans	118 grams	12.5 grams
Kidney Beans	118 grams	11.6 grams
Lentils	118 grams	12.1 grams
Lima Beans	118 grams	14.2 grams
Navy Bean	118 grams	18.1 grams
Pinto Beans	118 grams	11.0 grams

Fruit	Serving Size	Net Carbs
Apple	1 apple	17.4 grams
Apricot	1 medium	2.9 grams
Banana	1 small	21.2 grams
Grapefruit	1 quarter	7.9 grams
Grapes	8 grapes	7.1 grams
Guava	1 medium	5.8 grams
Kiwi	1 kiwi	8.7 grams
Mango	236 grams	87 grams
Nectarine	1 medium	13.8 grams
Papaya	½ cup	6.1 grams
Passion Fruit	60 grams	7.7 grams
Peach	1 small	7.2 grams
Pineapple	85 grams	8.7 grams
Plum	1 plum	7.6 grams
Tangerine	1 small	6.2 grams
Watermelon	118 grams	5.2 grams

Vegetables	Serving Size	Net Carbs
Acorn Squash	120 grams	7.6 grams
Beetroot	85 grams	6.8 grams
Butternut Squash	100 grams	7.9 grams
Carrots	177 grams	10.0 grams
Corn on the Cob	1 ear	17.2 grams
Jerusalem Artichoke	75 grams	11.9 grams
Parsnip	80 grams	10.8 grams
Swede	85 grams	5.9 grams
Sweet Potato	½ medium potato	9.9 grams
White Potato	118 grams	13.9 grams

Phase Four Acceptable Foods

By the time you reach Phase Four there are only a few foods that are yet to be included in your diet. These are highly starchy foods but are also pretty healthy for you. At this point your diet should be well under hand and you should need to make minimal adjustments in order to maintain your weight loss. Your meal plans should now be your new way of eating and you'll round it all out with these Phase Four additions.

Brown Rice	59 grams	10.2 grams
Oatmeal	118 grams	10.6 grams
Whole Wheat Pasta	59 grams	8.2 grams

While this list is extensive, it is in no way exhaustive. Every region of the world has specific foods that are unique to them so it would be impossible to list them all. If the food you're interested in is not on this list, remember just a few basic rules that will help you to decide if you should eat it or not.

In Phase 1 of the diet, you are given a wide range of foods to choose from but you'll notice that all the foods on the list have very little carbs if any. If you're in Phase 1 and 2, make sure that the foods you consume do not exceed 7 grams per serving. This way it'll be easier for you to stay within your daily carb limit. In Phases 3 and 4, you can be a little freer with your carbs but always stay within the range allowed for your limit.

Since everyone's body responds to food differently, you'll need to monitor your progress carefully. By doing so, it will be much easier for you to lose the weight and keep it off in the long term. Still, knowing which foods to eat and measuring portion sizes is only half the challenge of weight loss. The other half is in knowing how to prepare them so that they are appealing, flavorful, and satisfying. This is where many people fail in their new meal plans. The following chapters will list recipes that will give you step by step guidance in how to prepare your foods so that you can stick to your new nutritional plans.

Foods to Avoid

Even though you now have a very extensive list of foods you can eat and the right portion sizes, it is also important to have a list of foods that you should avoid at all costs. These foods are extremely high in carbohydrates and offer very little, if any, nutritional value for you to pull from. By avoiding these foods, you will avoid the risk of overreaching your Net Carb Count and be able to maintain your new routine.

White Bread: This does not mean that you have to eliminate all bread from your diet, but white bread in any form, should be avoided at all costs. It falls in the category of simple carbs and provides no real nutrition to support your new eating habits. Other breads can be included in Phases 2, 3, and 4 of your program as long as they have 1.8 grams of net carbs or less per serving.

Grains: These are often high in carbs and should be avoided for obvious reasons. However, once you reach Phase 4 you can eat these in small portion sizes as long as they don't push you over your carb allowance. These include grains like barley, wheat, spelt, rye, etc.

Pasta: Regular pasta is also very high in carbs and will not work well with a low carb diet. However, if you're a true pasta lover, you can once again enjoy it in your meals once you reach Phase 4. Just make sure it's whole wheat pasta and has less than 19 grams of net carbs per serving.

Diet and Low-Fat Foods: They may sound like they are good for you but in reality, these foods usually contain high amounts of sugars and preservatives that can send you over your carb limit.

Sugar based Sauces: If you must use sauces for your meals, make sure that you make them yourself. Many store bought sauces have added sugars not to mention the ingredients themselves have their own source of sugar. Look in the recipe chapter for a homemade tomato sauce that will taste just as good if not better than those supermarket brands, and it'll be more satisfying for you overall.

Cookies, Cakes, and Candies: Let's face it junk food is junk. These foods are very high in sugar content and will only complicate your efforts to stay on your program. The simple carbs they contain will be digested far too quickly to keep you satisfied, which is the complete opposite of what you hope to achieve.

Soft Drinks: While some may believe that soft drinks are the new water, they would be wrong. When you drink a can of soda, you're really consuming a beverage that is almost entirely made of sugar. It's true, these drinks do carry a bunch of flavor so if you need to drink something that has a little more flavor than water, try squeezing some juice into a bottle of mineral water. You'll drastically reduce the amount of sugar you consume but you'll get the same effect.

Now that you know the basics, it's time to get started on creating your meal plans.

CHAPTER 4

Creating Meal Plans

I t is one thing to have a list of foods to eat but it's another thing entirely to learn how to plan a meal so that it has enough energy to sustain you until the next meal, is emotionally satisfying, and will provide you with the essential nutrients your body needs. For the average person, this is a tall order. It is difficult to choose the right combination of foods, the best way to prepare them, and have enough variety in their diet that they don't get bored or discouraged after only a short period of time.

Remember, this meal program will be the start of a new life long way to eat, so you want to have as much variety as you can have and try to be as creative as possible to help you to stick with it for the long haul. Below are a few suggestions that can help you to get started creating your own meals. You don't have to follow these plans rigidly, if one food is not available in your area feel free to substitute with something else of equal nutritional value and above all else, it is essential that you do not exceed your net carb requirements for the day.

Breakfast Meal Plans

One of the biggest reasons why people fail to follow through with creating breakfast meal plans is a lack of time. If you're one of those who reaches for the box of cereal or the pop tart that you can just drop in the toaster and munch on it on the way out the door, you're probably feeling a little anxiety about this point. However, there are ways to prepare a healthy breakfast meal without having to spend a lot of time in the kitchen. Here are a few suggestions that can help to get your creative juices flowing.

Repurpose Leftovers: One of the easiest ways to get your motor going in the morning is to reheat leftovers from dinner the night before. You already know that the food will be within your allowable range and won't break your meal plan. Try preparing an extra portion when you are cooking your dinner and save it for your morning rush.

Leftover dinner vegetables can be great to add in a morning omelet to get you going in a rush.

Prepare the Ingredients The Night Before: For those who just have to have a real prepared breakfast, take the time to prepare the ingredients the day before so all you have to do is throw it together in the pan. This also works well for those who love to start their morning with a protein shake or a juice. If the ingredients are already cut, chopped, sliced, and ready to go all you have to do is throw them in the blender, push a button, and you're already off to a good start.

Prepare Ahead of Time: There are many breakfast meals that can be prepared ahead of time that can be refrigerated or frozen until ready to eat.

Eggs: You can scramble a large batch of them and portion them out. Cooked eggs can be stored in the fridge for 2-3 days and kept in the freezer for longer. They may not have the same consistency when thawed out but the nutritional value and benefits will still be there.

Flax Bread: This makes a great toast and is easy to prepare. Just sprinkle it with cheese and melt in the microwave. If you have time, add a little chopped bacon and top with a fried egg (or 2) and you're good to go.

Muffins: Great for the bread lover in the house. Prepare a batch of low-carb muffins ahead of time. On your way out the door, grab a little cottage cheese for protein and sprinkle a little cinnamon on it and you've got your protein boost to get your busy morning started.

Pancakes: If you're one of those people who loves to have pancakes in the morning, you'll be happy to know that they can also be made ahead of time and frozen until you're ready to use them. Serve them with sugar-free syrup or jam to sweeten them up a bit. If you really want to be creative try using peanut or almond butter as a spread instead. If you don't even have time for that, take two pancakes and use them as sandwich bread and fill it with your favorite protein. It's one of the fastest ways to make a breakfast you can live with.

Tips on Making Breakfast Fast

In many cases, it's impossible to prepare a breakfast without having to cook it. Finding the time to do this means you'll have to take a few shortcuts to get it done in the time allotted. But don't worry, you might even have fun learning a few of these little tricks.

The Pan Flip: When frying eggs in a pan you can waste a lot of time finding utensils, using them, and the cleaning them up later. Learning how to flip eggs in a pan cuts out a lot of those steps. Get yourself a non-stick pan and add a little spray oil and add your eggs. When they're cooked on one side and ready to be flipped, pick the pan up, give it a little swirl, tilt the pan downward at a 45 degree angle, flip it upwards and watch your egg flip. It'll take a little practice but you'll be amazed at how much time you'll save. Rather than 10 minutes to prepare your breakfast you'll spend only 2.

Microwave Your Eggs: Another way you can save time is preparing your eggs in the microwave. This works great for scrambled eggs. Prep your eggs just as you would if you were going to cook them on the stove top but instead put them in a microwavable dish and set it for 2 or 3 minutes. You can busy yourself with other things while your eggs are cooking.

Make Breakfast Wraps: If you're really on the run, take your breakfast ingredients and wrap them in a low-carb tortilla. You can fix them up any way you like as long as you don't exceed your net carb limit and stay within the recommended portion sizes.

The Non-Cook Breakfast: If you don't have any time at all to cook, then you can always reach for those non-cook items to start your day. These can include a cup of yogurt, a hunk of cheese, fruit, nuts, or seeds. It's important to note that you can only reach for these things if they are on your acceptable foods list for the Phase you're on.

Shakes: When making breakfast shakes, add a spoon of protein powder or soft tofu to give you that extra boost. If you choose to use protein powder, make sure you read the label carefully to be sure that the powder is not adding extra carbohydrates to your diet. Some powders carry as much as 40 grams of carbohydrates in one spoonful! Yikes! This will shatter your efforts to lose weight so choose carefully.

The Weekly Plan

Now that we've mastered the fundamentals of the low carb high fat diet, it is time for us to get down to creating the actual diet plan to follow. Keep in mind that your ultimate goal is to eat as much as possible and still lose weight. The meal plans that follow should be used as guides to give you ideas on how to accomplish that. The information is based on research and testimonials from a variety of people who've already tried these meals and have been successful. All you have to do is follow the guidelines laid out here and you will begin to see the results in a short time.

This chapter consists of a complete diet plan for seven days that will help you to get the most out of your low carb high fat diet routine. It should be noted that it is only a sample plan that you should feel free to "tweak" to meet your unique needs and requirements. However, it is important that any adjustments you make should still remain with the Acceptable Foods List for that phase and that you take care not to include any foods on the avoid list in your plan.

These meal plans are not all ideally suited for the Induction Phase of the diet so you will have to modify it for the phase you're on - always remembering that you need to consume more fats and keep the consumptions of carbs at its lowest possible point.

Since this is a new concept for most people it pays to have a plan to get into this new way of eating. Start with a "Ditch Day." This will be the day that you eliminate all the "avoid foods" from your home. Clean out your fridge and cupboards to reduce temptation. Keep in mind that you'll probably feel a bit sluggish while your metabolism adjusts to your new diet but after that you'll slide right into this new eating routine quite easily.

The next day we'll call the "Oil Change Day." This is the day when you'll change all the oils in your home to those healthy fats: coconut oil, olive oil, butter (the real kind, not the margarine), cream, cheese, avocado, coconut milk/cream, and the skins on your meat and fish (no need to avoid them now).

The following day, you can call the "Restock Day." You'll replace all processed foods with healthier options. Canned or jarred sauces will be replaced with your own homemade ones. Anything preprocessed should be removed from your house and replaced with all natural foods. Also you want to stock up on spices and seasonings. They won't add carbs to your meals but they'll definitely make the meals more appealing.

When restocking, make sure that you have plenty of things that will go bad in a short time. If flavor is not an incentive to eat them, the loss of the money certainly will. Stock up on vegetables when they are in season, meat, and fish and you won't go wrong.

Monday

Breakfast

Yogurt

Berries in cream with nuts and seeds

Lunch

Chicken Salad

Dinner

Salmon filet

Pumpkin mash

Asian vegetables

Snack

10 almonds

or 3 squares of dark chocolate

Tuesday

Breakfast

Cheesy scrambled eggs

Lunch

Crackers

Seed crackers

And vegetable platter

Dinner

Courgetti Bolognese

Snack

Apple slices with nut butter

Wednesday

Breakfast

Eggs and Bacon

Lunch

Leftover Bolognese

Salad with Cheese

Dinner

Asparagus

Feta Cheese Frittata

Snack

10 Almonds

Glass of wine

Low Carb High Fat

Thursday

Breakfast

Omelette

Lunch

Leftover Frittata

Dinner

Burger con todo

(substitute lettuce leaf for the bun)

Snack

3 squares of dark chocolate

Low Carb High Fat

Thursday

Breakfast
Omelette

Lunch
Leftover Frittata

Dinner
Burger con todo

(substitute lettuce leaf for the bun)

Snack
3 squares of dark chocolate

46

Friday

Breakfast

Coconut cream smoothie

Lunch

Tuna Super Salad

Dinner

Chicken curry with a faux rice

Snack

Apple slices with nut butter

Glass of wine

Saturday

Breakfast

Eggs with mushrooms and spinach

Lunch

Roasted Jerusalem Artichokes

With Garlicky Kale

Dinner

Russian Kale Squash Noodles

Snack

Avocado and Cacao Smoothie

Sunday

Breakfast

Simple Salad

With Lemony Almond Cheese

Lunch

Broccoli Salad

Dinner

Winter Kale Vegetable Stew

With Rutabaga Noodles

Snack

Avocado Chocolate Chip Cookies

Again, it is important to understand that these meal plans are simply guidelines. You do not have to restrict your diet to these basic dishes. Doing so would create a diet that will quickly get boring and you will lose interest. You are about to embark on a new life change so it's important that you make it what you want it to be.

A low carb high fat lifestyle needs to be appealing in order to be successful. While other diets encourage a "cheat day" doing so on this diet will delay your body's adjustment to the new changes. So, the more interesting you make your meals the less inclined you'll be to want to cheat.

Finally, as you pass through each phase of the program, you'll be allowed to eat more and more. By making the needed substitutions you'll find you won't miss many of your favorite foods. Consider these suggestions.

Foods to Avoid	Substitutions
Breakfast cereals	Nuts and seeds (No grain)
Rice	Faux rice (see recipe)
Potatoes or starchy vegetables	Faux potato, low carb vegies
Spaghetti/pasta	Cougetti or eggplant
Bread	Lettuce leaves
Crackers, biscuits, cake (etc.)	Seed crackers (see recipe)

In time, with your creativity you'll begin to come up with your own substitutions and once you get the hang of it, you'll find that this is probably the easiest diet program of them all.

CHAPTER 5

Breakfast Recipes

O k. You probably cringed when you saw that breakfast in the last chapter started with a bowl of yogurt and some berries. Well, I'm glad you stayed with us for the remainder because remember, that is only a suggestion of what to include in your diet. If you're accustomed to a more substantial meal to start the day it is certainly within the realm of possibilities. Try these recipes on for size:

Skillet Baked Eggs on a Bed of Spinach, with Yogurt

If eggs are your thing, then this dish will provide a perfect morning twist on your breakfast favorite. You won't even have to use a plate to serve it because you can eat it right out of the pan.

Ingredients

2/3 cup Greek yogurt (plain)

1 clove of garlic

Kosher salt

2 Tablespoons of butter (unsalted)

2 Tablespoons of olive oil

3 Tablespoons of chopped leeks (both parts)

2 Tablespoons chopped scallions (white and pale green, no dark parts)

10 cups of fresh spinach

1 teaspoon of fresh lemon juice

4 large eggs

¼ teaspoon of chili powder or ¼ teaspoon red pepper flakes

Pinch of paprika

1 teaspoon chopped oregano

Preparation

Mix yogurt, garlic, and salt in a small bowl and set aside to rest.

Preheat oven to 300 degrees.

Melt 1 Tablespoon of the butter together with the olive oil in a large heavy oven-proof skillet over medium heat. Add in the leeks and the scallions. Lower the heat and cook until they are soft. This should take about 10 minutes.

Mix in the spinach and lemon juice and salt to taste.

Increase the heat to a medium-high temperature and cook the spinach until it begins to wilt. This should take about 4-5 minutes.

Drain off the excess liquid. Make 4 holes in the spinach and carefully break one egg in each indentation, making sure not to burst the yolks. Place the pan in the oven and bake until the eggs set. This should take about 15 minutes.

Melt the remaining butter in a saucepan over medium heat. Add in the chili powder, salt, and cook until the butter begins to foam and begins to brown. Add in the oregano and let cook for about a half a minute longer before removing from heat.

Remove the garlic from the yogurt mixture and discard. Spoon the yogurt over the spinach and eggs and drizzle the spiced butter over it before serving.

This recipe serves 2-4 people

Cinnamon Faux Oatmeal

This recipe is not only perfect for the low carb/high fat diet it is also gluten free. The good part is that it's not really oatmeal but it's a combination of seeds and flax meal instead. A great substitute for a low carb breakfast boost. And you can make a batch of it and have it on hand so that the next time you need a quick breakfast it'll be ready.

Ingredients

½ cup of Chia seeds

½ cup of flax meal

½ cup of unsweetened coconut (finely shredded)

1¾ teaspoons of ground cinnamon

Preparation

Combine the chia seeds, flax meal, coconut, and cinnamon together and store in an airtight container.

To Serve

Scoop out ½ cup of the "faux" oatmeal mixture and pour in a bowl. Keep the remainder stored in the airtight container.

Pour ½ cup of hot water over the mixture and let sit for 5 minutes.

Sweeten to taste and add 2 Tablespoons of cream.

Stir to combine.

Add in fresh berries or toasted coconut for added texture and flavor.

Serve.

Simple Salad With Lemony Almond Cheese

For those who need to stay away from the eggs and the grains, this is another way to perk up your morning meal. Who says you have to have all those things in your breakfast? The Lemony Almond Cheese in this recipe is not really cheese at all.

Ingredients

1 cup of blanched almonds

1 teaspoon of sweet miso paste

¼ teaspoon of dulse (a dark red edible seaweed)

Yeast (optional)

Salad

Choose any mild leafy green

Grape tomatoes

Chopped red onions

A drizzle of lemon juice

Preparation

Place almonds in the food processor with just enough water so that they can be processed to a smooth texture.

Add in the dulse and miso paste.

Add a dash of yeast if you want.

Transfer the paste to a strainer lined with cheesecloth and let sit over a bowl to drain.

Place the bowl in a warm location and let rest overnight.

After around 12 hours taste the cheese to see if it has fermented long enough.

If so, wrap the cheese in the cheesecloth and shape the cheese into whatever shape you like and refrigerate to ripen.

If it needs more time, put it back in the warm place and wait a while longer.

Serve

Create the salad from the above vegetables and crumble the "faux" cheese over the top and serve.

Eggs in a Cloud

This recipe calls for the use of egg whites as a substitute for the starchier foods we tend to have for breakfast.

Ingredients

4 eggs

¼ cup of grated Romano (a hard salty-Italian cheese)

¼ cup chopped chives

¼ cup crumpled bacon

Ground black pepper

Preparation

Separate the egg whites from the yolks.

Place the yolks in 4 separate small bowls.

Whip the whites together until they form stiff peaks.

Fold in the cheese, along with the chives and bacon.

On a parchment lined baking sheet spoon the whites into four mounds

Make an indentation in the center of each mound.

Bake at 450 degrees for 3 minutes.

Add 1 yolk in each mound.

Season with salt pepper

Bake until the egg yolks set.

This should take about 2-3 minutes.

Gluten-Free Cinnamon and Coconut Pancakes

These may not taste like the traditional pancake recipe you're used to but there's a good chance you're going to like them better.

Ingredients

2 large eggs

3 Tablespoons of coconut milk **(full fat only)**

½ of a ripe banana (mashed)

½ teaspoon of apple cider vinegar

½ teaspoon of vanilla extract

1½ teaspoon of organic coconut flour

½ teaspoon cinnamon

¼ teaspoon baking soda

Pinch of salt

Coconut oil

Preparation

Blend the eggs, coconut milk, banana, vinegar, and vanilla together until thoroughly combined.

In a separate bowl mix the remaining ingredients leaving out only the coconut oil, which is reserved for frying.

Mix the wet and dry ingredients together just before cooking

Heat 1 Tablespoon of coconut oil over medium heat in a cast iron skillet.

Add a Tablespoon of batter.

When bubbles begin to form on the surface, flip the pancake over and let it cook for about 30 seconds on the other side.

Repeat for as many pancakes as you need or until you run out of batter.

Serve

These pancakes don't really need a topping but you can add your favorite fruit if you like.

Spinach and Ricotta Pie With Sausage Crust

This recipe is a great low carb way to start the day. While it calls for spinach you can substitute any green, leafy vegetable that you have around the house. And if you have your own garden you can't go wrong with throwing a bunch of your own handiwork into this dish. For those in phases where cheese is not on your acceptable foods, you can omit or use a comparable substitute.

Ingredients

1 Tablespoon olive oil

½ cup chopped onion

1 clove garlic (minced)

1 cups of ricotta cheese (whole milk)

3 eggs

1 cup of mozzarella (shredded)

¼ cup Parmesan (shredded)

1/8 teaspoon of ground nutmeg

Salt and pepper

1 lb. sausage (mild, medium, or hot)

Preparation

Heat the olive oil in a large skillet and add in onions and garlic. Cook until the vegetables are tender. Add in the spinach (or your choice of greens) and cook until the leaves begin to wilt. Add in the nutmeg and other seasonings.

Remove from heat and let cool

In a large bowl beat the eggs. Mix in the three cheeses and stir until well blended.

Stir in the cooked spinach.

You can make smaller individual pies or you can make one large one. If you're planning on the larger pie, roll out your sausage meat and press into your pie tin until it is even all the way around. If making individual pies, use a muffin tin instead.

Pour in the mixture and place on a cookie sheet (this will keep the fats from the sausage from dripping on to the bottom of your oven).

Bake at 350 degrees F until the sausages are firm.

This should take about 30 minutes.

Remove from the oven and serve hot!

Stuffed Bell Peppers

This dish is a great way to spice up your breakfast in the mornings. If you have the time, you can do this for the whole family. They will love it!

Ingredients

½ lb. chorizo

½ onion (chopped)

2 cloves of garlic (minced)

6 eggs

¼ cup whole milk (or substitute)

½ cup mozzarella cheese (shredded)

Chopped fresh parsley

3 bell peppers with the tops cut off and seeded

Salt and pepper

Preparation

Pre-heat over to 350 degrees (F)

Brown the chorizo in a large skillet

Add onion and garlic and mix well.

Cook for about 3 minutes.

In a separate bowl whisk together the eggs, milk, cheese, parsley, salt and pepper.

Add in the cooked chorizo and blend well.

Pour the mixture into the bell pepper cavity and place in a baking dish.

Bake until the egg are cooked through (about 35-40 minutes)

Top with the bell pepper tops.

Serve.

CHAPTER 6

Lunch Recipes

Most people are often busy when lunchtime rolls around. If you're one of those, you won't have a lot of time to break away to fix a good meal so you will have to be smart about your food preparation. Here are a few simple ideas that you can piggyback on when it's time for your midday meal. They are simple and with just a few adjustments, you'll find that lunchtime can be one of the best times to give yourself a little boost of energy.

Low Carb Chicken Salad

Chicken salad is one of the most convenient foods you can have when you're on a low carb diet. You can perk it up in a wide range of ways and you don't even have to worry about going over your carb count. Whether you're on the Induction Phase or you've reach all the way to the end of the program just a few tweaks to an old favorite can give you a fabulous meal that you can't possibly go wrong with.

Ingredients

2 cups of cooked chicken (shredded)

1 stalk of celery (sliced very thin)

3 green onions (chopped)

¼ cup of pecans (or another preferred nut on your list) chopped

1 Tablespoon of minced dill

1 cup of homemade mayonnaise

2 Tablespoons of hot mustard

Salt and pepper

Preparation

Toss celery, onions, and chicken in a large bowl

In a separate bowl, mix together the mayonnaise, pecans, hot mustard, salt and pepper

Add dill and any of your favorite herbs for flavoring

Pour the mayonnaise dressing over the chicken mixture and mix thoroughly.

Refrigerate for 2-3 hours before serving.

Makes 4 servings

Gluten Free Seed Crackers

It can be hard to let go of some of our favorites and bread and crackers seem to be the most craved foods once the low carb diet has begun. If crackers have been some of your favorite foods, then you're probably already missing them. Here is a great substitute for an old time favorite that you'll be able to reach for anytime you get that urge for something with a little crack to it.

Ingredients

½ cup of sunflower seeds

½ cup of pumpkin seeds

¼ cup of sesame seeds

¼ cup of poppy seeds

¼ cup of flaxseed

¼ cup of Chia seeds

½ teaspoon salt

1 cup water

Sea salt

Preparation

Preheat oven to 350 degrees.

Place all the seeds and salt in a bowl

Pour in water and mix until combined

Let stand for 15 minutes while the Chia and flaxseeds soften and stick together.

Pour seeds out on a cookie sheet lined with baking paper

Spread mixture out as thin as possible

Sprinkle with sea salt

Bake for 30 minutes

Remove from oven and slice into small crackers.

Return to the oven and cook for an additional 30 minutes or until crisp and golden brown.

Remove from oven and let cool.

Store in an airtight container until ready to eat.

Tuna Super Salad

What's great about this recipe is that it is loaded with lots of low carb veggies so you can pretty much eat as much as you want. If one serving doesn't fill you up, feel free to have another and another and another. Another great thing about this is that it can be your own creation, you can go crazy and nothing will happen to you. All you need to do is top it off with your favorite protein. If tuna is not your thing, substitute chicken or some other protein so that your meal has enough substance to carry you through the rest of the day.

Ingredients

Choose your own leafy green. Lettuce of course is the popular choice but even there you'll have lots of variety.

Add in a bunch of chopped veggies. You can add as many as you like but make sure you pick those low carb ones so you can have your fill. Suggestions could be beets, carrots, jicama, celery, cucumber, cauliflower, snow peas, and tomatoes. Try to choose those that are in season so you'll have plenty of them.

Choose your protein. You can make this a real meal by giving it substance. This recipe calls for tuna but you can change that to whatever you like; tofu, chickpeas, eggs. Make it whatever you prefer.

Choose a fat. Remember this is a diet you can have a little fat with. It will help you to feel satisfied and can help the body to absorb all the nutrients you're getting with all those delicious veggies you've built up. You can pretty much choose whatever you want but some suggestions are avocado slices, olives, nuts, or seeds if they're not on your avoid list.

Now, make your dressing. Dressings pretty much have the same basic components; a base could be vinaigrette, cream, or soy sauce are just a few suggestions. Then add in a little garlic, lemon juice, and other flavorings to give it a little bite. Oil based dressings can use olive, canola, grapeseed, or safflower oil. Mix it with the spices and a little vinegar.

Finally you want to add a little texture to make sure that you get the satisfaction you can only get from chewing. Dried fruit (cranberries or raisins), pita chips, nuts, etc.

Note on Super Salads: These salads can be amazing meals in and of themselves. They are rich in all the nutrients and using fresh greens and veggies make them some of the most healthiest meal choices you can have. That said; avoid using pre-packaged ingredients. Whenever possible go with fresh veggies all the way. It's not hard to make your own dressing. Once you get the hang of it you won't want to buy store bought ever again.

Roasted Jerusalem Artichokes

Artichokes can be a great way to add a new texture to the old flavors. They are a delicate food but rich in nutritious value and they work well with the low carb diet plan.

Ingredients

1 lb. of chopped Jerusalem artichokes

1 chopped parsnip

1 bell pepper chopped

3 cloves of garlic, chopped

½ teaspoon salt

¼ teaspoon ground black pepper

1 Tablespoon of vegetable oil

Fresh parsley

Preparation

Preheat the oven to the lowest temperature.

Spread the artichokes, parsnip, and the bell pepper out on a baking sheet

Toss in the garlic and season with salt and pepper

Drizzle with oil and use your hands to mix it all together.

Make sure that everything has a light coat of oil.

Slow roast it in the oven until the vegetables are nice and tender

Transfer to a plate and garnish with fresh parsley

Garlicy Kale

You can make your own dressing if you like. It is simple and easy to do and won't take a lot of time.

Ingredients

2 Tablespoons of vegetable oil

1 large onion, chopped fine

4 garlic cloves, minced

2 bunches of kale, remove stems and chop

Salt and pepper

Nutmeg

¼ cup of vegetable stock

Preparation

Heat the oil in a large pan over medium high heat.

Add the onions and cook until they are translucent

Add in the garlic and mix well.

Cook until the aromas are released

Add in the kale a little at a time.

Toss with the salt, pepper, and a pinch of nutmeg.

As the kale slowly wilts continue to add more until you have added it all.

Pour in the stock

Turn the heat down to low, cover and allow it to cook until the kale has turned to a bright green color.

Serve while it is still hot.

Broccoli Salad

This recipe only takes 10 minutes to make so if you're looking for a quick lunch you won't have to worry about getting back to business when you need to. You can even prepare this salad ahead of time and refrigerate it until you're ready for it. It's delicious and is packed with lots of nutrition too.

Ingredients

6 cups of uncooked broccoli

½ onion chopped

1 cup of homemade mayonnaise

½ cup of chopped almonds

2 Tablespoons of red vinegar

8 slices of bacon, precooked and chopped

salt and pepper

Preparation

Combine the broccoli, bacon, onion, and almonds together in a large bowl

Toss until well mixed

In a separate bowl blend together the mayonnaise, vinegar, salt and pepper

Pour the dressing over the broccoli mixture and stir until all the ingredients are evenly coated.

Cover and refrigerate for an hour or more

Serve cold.

Roasted Spaghetti Squash with Basil and Parmesan

If you're longing for a little pasta but are afraid of the carbs try this recipe and you won't miss your pasta again. Spaghetti squash is about as close as you're going to get to the real deal but it packs lots of vitamin A, B, and C into each bite. Add to that a bunch of minerals like calcium, magnesium, manganese, and potassium and you have an awesome super food that will definitely help you get your energy back so you can finish the day.

Ingredients

One medium sized spaghetti squash

1½ Tablespoon of coconut oil

Salt and pepper

1 Tablespoon of fresh squeezed lemon juice

½ teaspoon of dried basil

¼ cup of Parmesan cheese (optional)

Preparation

Preheat the oven to 375 degrees

Cut the spaghetti squash lengthwise and remove the seeds

Brush the inside with melted coconut oil

Sprinkle the squash with salt and pepper

Turn upside down on a baking sheet lined with parchment paper

Roast in the oven for 45 minutes or until the squash is soft and tender

Take a fork and shred the flesh of the squash

In a separate bowl, mix together the lemon juice and basil with coconut oil

Toss the spaghetti squash in the mixture

Top with Parmesan cheese and serve.

Fritatta With Bacon and Asparagus

Frittatas can be cooked in a very short amount of time so they can be a great low-carb menu option. One of the great things about frittatas is that they keep well so you can make it ahead of time and pack it for your lunch.

Ingredients

2 eggs

Sea salt

Ground pepper

Seasonings of your choice

Handful of grilled asparagus spears

Olive oil

Bacon pieces

1 teaspoon of Parmesan cheese

Preparation

Take the asparagus spears and lay them out on a baking sheet drizzled with olive oil.

Bake in oven for 20 minutes at 350 degrees

While the asparagus is baking

Beat the eggs with the salt, pepper, and other seasonings

Add in the precooked asparagus spears, bacon pieces, and Parmesan cheese.

Cook together in a heavy skillet until the bottom has set.

Finish preparing in the oven until the eggs are all fully set.

Serve with avocado slices as a garnish or a side salad.

CHAPTER 7

Dinner Recipes

D inners can be one of the best times for you to enjoy your meals and get the most satisfaction out of every bite. People tend to have more time at dinner so they can sit back and really take the time to relax and unwind while they are eating. Still, there are some who may not have the time for that. We live very busy lives so being balanced is necessary.

With a practical approach to your dinner time meals you can make a double portion of these meals and have them for lunch the next day, mix them up a bit and have a little for snacks throughout the day. Take these recipes as a guide to stir up your creative juices, experiment with them, and change them around a bit. Before long, you'll find that you have created your own recipe ideas that you can share with others so that they can also enjoy the benefits of the low carb/high fat nutrition program.

Grilled Salmon Filet with a Pumpkin Mash and Asian Style Vegetables

One of the great things about salmon is that it is loaded with nutrition, high in protein, omega-3 fatty acids, and a little vitamin D to boot. It is the perfect food for the low carb high fat diet because it's easy to make, doesn't take a lot of time, and it's delicious.

Grilled Salmon Ingredients

Olive oil cooking spray

¾ teaspoon of sea salt

¾ teaspoon of freshly ground black pepper

1 pint of cherry tomatoes cut in half

2 Tablespoons of extra-virgin olive oil

2 Tablespoons of balsamic vinegar

3 Tablespoons of basil, sliced thin and a few whole basil sprigs

4 4-ounce salmon fillets

Preparation

Put tomatoes, olive oil, vinegar, and sliced basil in a bowl

Season with ¼ teaspoon each of salt and pepper

Let sit at room temperature for at least 15 minutes before serving over the salmon filets

Grilled Salmon Filets

Lightly coat both sides of the salmon filets with the olive oil cooking spray

Use the remaining ¼ teaspoon each of salt and pepper to season.

Place the filets skin side down on the grill and cook 3 or 4 minutes or until they turn a nice golden brown.

Turn and cook for 3 more minutes on the other side.

Fish should be slightly firm in the center (if you use a thermometer, it should be 145 degrees when inserted)

Remove salmon and place on plates to serve.

Top with tomato relish (above)

Pumpkin Mash

This can be a great way to replace everybody's favorite mashed potatoes, which are usually loaded with carbs, and still get a great dish that everyone will enjoy.

Ingredients

1 small pumpkin, peeled and cleaned

¼ cup coconut cream

½ cup grated Parmesan

2 teaspoons minced garlic

2 teaspoons of sea salt

¼ teaspoon of freshly ground black pepper

Preparation

Wash the pumpkin and let dry.

Cut off a thin slice of the stem end and cut the pumpkin in half

Use an ice cream scoop to remove the seeds and the pulp

(You can reserve the seeds and roast them later for a great snack)

Cut the pumpkin into 1-inch cubes

Place the cubes in a large, glass bowl and cover with cling wrap.

Place in microwave and cook on high for 15 minutes stopping on occasion to stir the pieces. They should be very tender when done with no firm spots.

Take half of the cooked pumpkin cubes and put in the food processor and finely chop.

Add the remaining pumpkin and blend it all together.

Blend in the coconut cream, Parmesan cheese, minced garlic, salt and pepper.

Process it all until very smooth. (About 1 minute) making sure to scrape the sides with a spatula as you go.

Serve with stir-fried or steamed Asian vegetables

Courgetti Bolognese

This dish is another great alternative to the high carb pastas that everyone seems to love. For the Bolognese, we use minced turkey to create a great low-calorie sauce.

Ingredients

2 Tablespoons of olive oil

18 ounces of minced turkey

1 large onion, finely chopped

1 garlic clove, crushed

2 large carrots, peeled and diced finely

5 ½ ounces of button mushrooms, chopped

1 Tablespoon of tomato puree

2 lbs. of chopped tomatoes

2 cups of chicken stock

4 large courgettes

Parmesan cheese

Fresh basil leaves

Preparation

Heat 1 Tablespoon of the olive oil in a large saucepan

Add the minced turkey meat and cook until browned.

Place in a bowl and set aside to rest.

Add onion to the pan and cook on a low heat until they are soft

Add the garlic, stirring continuously for 1 minute

Add the carrots and the mushrooms, continuing to stir for an additional 3 minutes.

Add the minced turkey back into the pan

Add the chopped tomatoes and let simmer until the tomatoes are soft

Pour in 2 cups of chicken stock and bring it all to a boil.

Lower the heat and simmer for about 1½ hours until the tomatoes have thickened into a sauce and all the vegetables are tender.

While the Bolognese is still cooking, blend together the remaining seasonings. Spiralize your courgettes and set aside

Heat up a large frying pan with 1 Tablespoon of olive oil

Add in the courgetti

Cook until they are just barely soft (2-3 minutes)

Mix in the seasoning

Plate the Courgetti and top with the Bolognese

Grate a little pecorino and basil leaves

Serve immediately

Chicken Curry With Faux Rice

This dish is very easy to make and is a favorite for many people. Make a double portion and have it for lunch the next day.

Ingredients

3 Tablespoons of butter

2 pounds of chicken breasts, cut into 1-inch strips

1 teaspoon of ground cumin

½ teaspoon dried coriander

½ teaspoon dried ginger

¼ teaspoon of crushed red pepper flakes

4 finely chopped garlic cloves

½ cup of chicken stock

1/3 cup of coconut cream

1 Tablespoon of chopped fresh cilantro

Preparation

Melt butter in a heavy casserole dish over medium-high heat until it the foaming of the butter starts to slow.

Add in chicken strips a little at a time until they are browned.

Add the cumin, coriander, ginger, garlic, and the red pepper flakes and cook until all the seasonings are mixed well (about 2 minutes)

Add the chicken stock and bring it all to a boil

Reduce heat and let simmer for about 5 minutes (stir occasionally.

Slowly blend in the coconut cream and continue to simmer (make sure it does not come to a boil)

Serve over faux rice

Faux Rice

Rice is a common staple in most homes so it can be difficult to give up. It serves as a base for many different foods and it is a great side dish for breakfast, lunch or dinner. So it's really great to find that you can actually make a low carb substitute that can be used in replacement for the traditional favorite. This recipe makes up to 10 servings and only has 3 grams of carbs per serving.

Ingredients

20 ounces of fresh cauliflower

Butter

Salt and pepper

Preparation

Trim off the leaves of the tough stalks of cauliflower

Chop the vegetable into pieces small enough to fit into the food of your food processor and set on grate.

Put the grated cauliflower into a 2 ½ quart casserole dish

Add 2-4 Tablespoons of water, cover and microwave on the high setting for 10 minutes.

Stir every 5 minutes and check to make sure it is has a tender texture that is not mushy.

Add butter and season with salt and pepper

Spaghetti Squash Noodles With Peanut Sauce

You can't get any better than this dish. This dish, although vegan, has enough substance to satisfy a hungry stomach and it is packed full of vitamins, nutrients, and proteins to make sure you're fully nourished by the time your plate is empty.

Squash Ingredients

1 large spaghetti squash – cut in half and seeded

4-5 stalks of kale, stems removed

1 shallot, peeled

½ cup of chopped toasted cashews (optional)

3 Tablespoons toasted sesame seeds

Cilantro

1 bunch of broccoli florets

Salt and pepper

Peanut Sauce Ingredients

½ inch fresh ginger, peeled and chopped

2 cloves of chopped garlic

1-2 teaspoons of hot sauce

2 Tablespoons of sunflower seed butter

1 lime, peeled and chopped

1 Tablespoon of rice vinegar

2 Tablespoons of honey

1.5 Tablespoons of soy sauce

Extra virgin coconut oil

Sesame oil

½ cup of grapeseed oil

Preparation

Preheat the oven to 375 degrees

Cover a baking sheet with parchment paper and place the 2 squash halves on it with the cut side down.

Bake until the flesh separates from the skin in strands.

Cut the kale leaves into 1/3-inch strips and place in a large bowl.

Cut the shallot in half lengthwise and slice them into thin half moons and set aside.

Chop the herbs and cashews and set aside.

Put about an inch of water in a medium sized saucepan over medium heat.

Bring to a slow boil.

Place the broccoli florets in a colander and set it over the simmering water to steam.

Mix all the sauce ingredients in a blender and blend well.

Taste to adjust seasonings and set aside.

Remove squash from the oven, scrape the strands out with a fork and mix in a large bowl with kale.

Pour the dressing into the bowl.

Season with salt and pepper and toss together.

Divide the squash noodles into 4 bowls.

Top each one with the steamed broccoli, shallots, nuts, sesame seeds, herbs, and remaining sauce.

Serve immediately

Winter Kale Vegetable Stew With Rutabaga Noodles

Making rutabaga noodles can be a challenge, so if you're not up to it, feel free to substitute them with spaghetti noodles. However, if you have the time to try the rutabaga, it'll be well worth your effort.

Ingredients

1 large rutabaga, peeled and trimmed into noodles

3 cups of kale

1 Tablespoon extra virgin olive oil

½ cup sweet onions, diced

3 cloves of garlic, minced

½ teaspoons of red pepper flakes

1 cup of carrots, diced

1 cup of celery, diced

1 lb. of diced tomatoes, seeded

2 cups of vegetable broth

1 teaspoon of dried thyme

1 teaspoon of dried oregano

1 bay leaf

Salt and pepper to taste

¼ cup of red wine

Preparation

Preheat the oven to 425 degrees.

Line a baking sheet with parchment paper and lay out your noodles.

Coat the noodles with cooking spray and season with salt and pepper.

Set aside.

Place a large pot over medium heat

Coat the inside with cooking spray and add in the kale

Cook until they begin to wilt, tossing regularly.

Place the cooked kale on a plate and set aside.

Return the pot to the stove on medium heat.

Pour in the olive oil to heat it.

Add in onions, garlic, pepper flakes, carrots, and celery.

Cook until the vegetables are soft, stirring frequently.

Add a few drops of water if you find that the vegetables are sticking to the pan.

Add the tomatoes, vegetable broth, thyme, oregano, bay leaf, red wine, cooked kale, and salt and pepper and stir well.

Cover and let it come to a boil.

Reduce the heat to low and allow it to simmer uncovered for 30 minutes.

Make sure that the vegetables are tender and the stew has thickened.

Place the rutabaga noodles in the oven for 20 minutes (or until al dente).

Portion into bowls and set aside.

Remove the bay leaf from the stew and spoon over the rutabaga noodles.

Garnish with a little Parmesan cheese (optional)

Serve.

Lamb Ribs With Herb Sauce

This dish might become so popular that you'll have to make it a regular weekly meal. The lamb offers a nice switch from the traditional beef, chicken, and pork and when it's cooked to perfection you won't even realize you're eating diet food.

Ingredients

2 lbs. of lamb ribs

1 ½ cup of vegetable beef stock

1 teaspoon of fresh thyme

Juice from 1 lemon

2 garlic cloves, crushed

Himalayan sea salt and black pepper

Herb Sauce Ingredients

1 teaspoon of chopped parsley

1 teaspoon of chopped coriander

1 teaspoon of chopped fresh oregano

1 spring onion, chopped very fine

1 Tablespoon of lemon juice

1/3 cup of extra virgin olive oil

Lemon wedges

Preparation

Preheat over to 350F

Cover a baking sheet with aluminum foil

Place ribs on the sheet

Pour the stock over the ribs

Sprinkle the thyme, lemon juice, and garlic and toss really well to coat the ribs.

Cover with a second piece of foil making sure to seal the edges to create a package.

Roast in the oven for 35 minutes

Remove top foil cover and increase oven temperature to 400F

Roast until ribs are a crispy golden brown

Herb Sauce

Mix all the herbs together and add in the spring onion.

Stir in lemon juice and olive oil.

Whisk the entire mixture until blended well.

Serve the ribs while they are still hot and top with herb sauce

Garnish with lemon wedges.

Rib-Eye Steak and Fried Tomatoes

Ingredients

4 10 oz. rib-eye steaks

2 Tablespoons of olive oil

1 lb. of cherry tomatoes

1 Tablespoon fresh rosemary, chopped

2 cloves of garlic, chopped

2 Tablespoons of capers, chopped

Salt and pepper

1 Tablespoon of butter

Zest from 1 lemon

1 Tablespoon of flat leaf parsley, chopped

Grated Parmesan cheese (optional)

Preparation

In a large frying pan, heat the olive oil and add in the tomatoes.

Cook them until the skins begin to burst

Add in the rosemary, garlic, and capers, and cook them through for six minutes

Add the salt and pepper to taste.

Slowly stir in the butter and zest and cook for one more minute.

Stir in the parsley and set aside until the steaks are done.

Season the steaks and fry them the way you like them.

Place one steak on each plate and top with the cooked tomatoes. (Reheat the tomatoes if you need to).

Serve with a side salad

Black Forest Ham With Spicy Nuts

This dish is another twist on an old tradition. It doesn't take long to prepare and is a great way to introduce new flavors and textures to your meal plan. The more variety you can have in your meals, the easier it will be to stick with it.

Ingredients

3 ½ ounces of Black Forest Ham

7 ounces of uncooked mixed nuts

1 Tablespoon of butter

1 Tablespoon of olive oil

1 teaspoon of ground cumin

1 teaspoon of paprika

Dash of cayenne pepper

Preparation

Preheat oven to 350 degrees F

Place the ham on a wire rack set over a baking sheet

Bake in the oven for 15 minutes or until the ham gets crispy

Cut the ham into small slices and set aside

Brown the nuts in a heavy pan over a low heat

Add the butter, olive oil, and spices.

Add the ham – make sure that the ham is fully coated with spices

Fry until it is a nice golden brown color

Line a separate baking sheet with paper towels

Heat the oven to 300 degrees F

Place nuts on the sheet and put in the oven for 10 minute

Serve as a side dish for the ham, or as a snack dish to much on during snack time.

CHAPTER 8

Snack Ideas

No matter what type of diet program you choose to be on, the biggest challenge that people have is snack time. There are lots of people who can eat healthy at every single meal of the day and lose it all with just one poor snack choice. The problem often lies in a lack of quality selections. Walk into any convenience store and you're immediately tempted with an array of high-sugar, high-carb, and high-fat choices. Healthier options, if any, are somewhere hidden along the back shelf where few customers dare to roam.

When you're on the low carb/high fat diet, you'll have to be extra careful about your snack choices. As a matter of fact, you'll probably soon realize that buying your snacks on the run will be out of the question. Your best bet to ensure that you don't exceed your daily carb allowance is to prepare your snacks ahead of time and always have something within arms reach to munch on when you get those cravings.

In the beginning of your diet, at the Induction Phase, you can almost count on those hunger pangs coming at the most inopportune time. Your body will have not yet gotten used to your new way of eating so it will be really helpful to have a few carb free snacks to help keep you satisfied. In the chapter on menu ideas, we listed a few simple ones. Chocolate squares, fruit slices, nuts and seeds are just some of the things you can have. But there will be times when you'll want a different texture, more substance, or just a different experience. Here are a few basic snack ideas you can try.

Smoothies

Our menu chapter calls for an **Avocado and Cacao Smoothie** but you can make just about any type of smoothie you want. They are rich with all the nutrients you need and if you add in just a small amount of protein powder, you'll also get a well-deserved energy boost whenever you need it. Here are some basic rules for making smoothies.

1. **Start with your liquid.** Choose something that fits within your acceptable foods list. Use about 1 or 2 cups but you can adjust it according to your liking. Some people prefer thicker smoothies. In that case, it's best to add a little liquid. Others prefer a more fluid texture, so you'll add more.

2. Recommended liquids for smoothies: water, almond milk, coconut milk, fruit juices, tea, or kefir. Whatever liquid you choose, it's important that you make sure it's on your acceptable foods list and that it doesn't take you over your carb allowance.

3. **Choose your base:** Every smoothie has a base. This is the ingredient that gives it that creamy texture or "body." Many smoothies will choose bananas for this because bananas blend very well and can become quite 'creamy' without a lot of effort. They also provide a natural sweetness. Other possibilities for bases are mangos, pears, peaches, apples, or avocados.

4. Make sure you avoid using water based fruits for the base as they won't help to create that texture that makes smoothies so appealing, so try not to use oranges, watermelons, or pineapples for bases.

5. **Flavors and Nutrients:** Your next step is to add the body of your smoothie. This is where you're going to create the perfect taste for your smoothie. Here you can experiment and turn on your creative juices. Choose from your fruits or vegetables list. Green smoothies are predominately made from green vegetables like beet greens, dandelion greens, arugula, kale, lettuce, or spinach. Fruit smoothies can also be thrown in too.

6. **Extras:** Finally, you can add in your extras. These can be your nuts, seeds, spices, protein powders, cacao, coconut meat, acai, or anything else that will boost the nutritional value of your smoothie.

7. **Blend:** Finally, blend it all together and you're ready to go. Smoothies can be a great way to have a quick pick-me-up when you're craving a snack, without having to risk jeopardizing your carb allowance.

Other Snack Ideas

Avocado Chocolate Chip Cookies

These little treats are easy to make and because they are flourless, they have a considerably low carb count.

Ingredients

3 ripe avocados, mashed

1 scoop of chocolate protein powder

1 ¼ cup of almond flour

¼ cup of flax meal

1/3 cup of sweetener (your choice)

5 Tablespoons of unsweetened coco powder (optional)

½ cup of unsweetened chocolate chips

1 teaspoon of baking powder

Preparation

Preheat the oven to 350 degrees F.

Spray coconut oil cooking spray on two baking sheets

Mix the mashed avocados and sweetener together in a large bowl.

Add the flour mixture to the mashed avocados. Make sure everything is fully incorporated.

Stir in the chocolate chips.

Place Tablespoon size balls of cookie dough on the baking sheet leaving about a 1½-inch space between them.

Flatten each cookie with a spatula

Bake for 10-12 minutes – you'll know when the edges have set.

Remove from oven and let cool.

Other Snack Ideas

1 ounce of string cheese

Celery stuffed with cream cheese

Cucumber slices with tuna or chicken salad

Beef or Turkey Jerky

Deviled Eggs

Lettuce leaf wraps with cheese

Green beans wrapped in ham slices

Sliced grilled tomatoes with basil and mozzarella cheese

Hummus with vegetables

Popcorn

Carrot sticks

And the list goes on.

Finally, Low Carb Sauces

We've already talked about great ways to substitute pastas but let's face it. No pasta is worth its salt if it doesn't have a good sauce to top it. Here is a suggested recipe for a low cost pasta sauce along with a barbecue sauce, and a pretty good pizza sauce.

Basic Tomato Sauce for Pasta

Ingredients

¼ cup of Extra virgin olive oil

1 medium onion, chopped

½ stalk of celery

2 cloves of garlic

1 teaspoon of dried basil

2 lbs. of tomatoes

Preparation

In a medium saucepan heat the olive oil over medium heat

Add the onions, celery, and garlic and cook until they are tender

Add the basil and continue to cook until well blended.

Stir in the tomatoes and allow the mixture to come to a boil.

Lower the heat to a simmer and leave the pan partially covered.

Cook the sauce until it begins to thicken.

Add salt and pepper to taste.

Serve over your favorite faux pasta.

Barbecue Sauce

This sauce will work great with almost any type of meat you choose and with only 3.7 net carbs per serving it can help you to join the crowd at any of the holiday festivities. You might even be surprised that everyone else will want to use your sauce instead of their own.

Ingredients

1 Tablespoon of Extra virgin olive oil

¼ cup of chopped onions

1 teaspoon of chili powder

1 teaspoon of cumin

¾ teaspoon of garlic powder

¾ teaspoon of hot mustard

¼ teaspoon of ground allspice

1/8 teaspoon of red pepper flakes

1½ cups of unsweetened ketchup

1 Tablespoon of apple cider vinegar

2/3 Tablespoon of Worcestershire Sauce

2 teaspoons of sugar substitute (optional)

¼ teaspoon of instant coffee

Note: Feel free to adapt these ingredients to your liking. If you prefer your sauce to be more tart, add more vinegar and hot mustard, if you like it a little on the sweet side, you can adjust the amount of sweetness.

Preparation

barbecue meat you prepare

Pizza Sauce

This sauce does not stray too far from the original so the taste will remain true to what you remember.

Ingredients

2 Tablespoons of Extra Virgin olive oil

1 teaspoon of minced garlic

½ cup of chopped onions

4 Tablespoons of tomato paste

1 teaspoon of basil leaves

¾ teaspoon of dried oregano

½ teaspoon of fennel seed

½ packet of sugar substitute (optional)

½ teaspoon of salt

¼ teaspoon of black pepper

¼ teaspoon of red pepper flakes

2 lbs. of fresh tomatoes (peeled and seeded)

Preparation

Heat olive oil in a medium saucepan over a medium heat

Add the crushed garlic and onions

Sauté until tender and translucent

Add the tomato paste, basil, oregano, fennel, sugar substitute, salt, pepper, and red pepper flakes.

Continue to cook while stirring

Add the tomatoes and continue to cook over medium heat until heated through.

Turn heat down to low and let simmer until it thickens.

Remove from heat and use immediately.

CONCLUSION

A low carb and high fat diet is a pretty authentic and reliable solution for achieving weight loss. Based on the testimonials from a large audience of people and the also the research conducted by many reliable scientists, it can be safely proposed that it can produce acceptable results.

The fact cannot be negated that obesity is becoming more and more common with the passage of time. Thus, there is a pressing need at this time to eradicate this prevalent problem. In this regard, the low carb and high fat diet is one of the most effective solutions. However, before following this plan – it is recommended that you consult your physician to avoid any issues.

Comprehensively, it can be stated that the results produced by this diet vary from person to person and the effectiveness can be different based on how the complete diet plan was executed.

Keeping all these considerations in mind, we have tried our best to provide you with the most reliable, valuable, and authentic knowledge. We hope that the information contained in this book will prove to be effective in producing results for you. However, it should be noted that you will only be able to see the results if you stay motivated, consistent, determined, and result-oriented throughout the whole process.

This said, we hope that you will exert yourself in implementing all the information contained in this book. Only successful execution of the plan can guarantee the results.

We wish you the best of luck, and all the happiness in this world!

Stay happy, and keep inspiring people around you.

Thank you again for downloading this book!

I hope this book was able to help you.

The next step is to check out my other books below!

Finally, if you enjoyed this book, then I'd like to ask you for a favor, would you be kind enough to leave a review for this book on Amazon? It'd be greatly appreciated!

Click here to leave a review for this book on Amazon!

Thank you and good luck!

About the Author

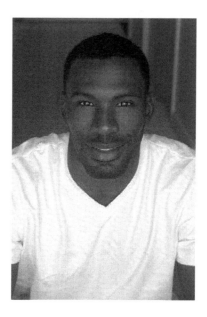

I am a health and fitness enthusiast that loves to teach people about losing weight and feeling better about themselves. I believe health and eating the right way is essential to your life in all aspects. For many years I have been studying different diet techniques and approaches to transform the human body. One of my biggest passions is helping others achieve the body that they have always wanted. I look forward to helping teach you how to be healthy and live a better life.

My goal is to publish books that will empower readers to improve their health and well-being through simple everyday ingredients and low fat recipes that make eating affordable, realistic, and delicious.

CHECK OUT MY OTHER BOOKS

Below you'll find some of my other popular books that are popular on Amazon and Kindle as well. Simply click on the links below to check them out. Alternatively, you can visit my author page on Amazon to see other work done by me.

HCG Diet - *http://amzn.to/1KRI1V1*

Dash Diet - *http://amzn.to/1IQ2tQ5*

Medittereanean Diet - *http://amzn.to/1IXhl0F*

Anti Inflammatory Diet - *http://amzn.to/1O3NgSB*

If the links do not work, for whatever reason, you can simply search for these titles on the Amazon website to find them.

Made in the USA
Middletown, DE
21 April 2018